MW01294988

66 Test Questions Student Respiratory Therapists Get Wrong Every Time... (Volume 1 of 2)

And Now You Don't Have Too!

Brady Nelson RRT

Forward by Graham Werstiuk RRT

VOLUME 1 FEATURES:

- 11 Patient Assessment Questions

- 11 Pulmonary Function Questions

- 11 Basic Science Questions

- 11 Cardiopulmonary Anatomy & Physiology Questions

- 11 Soft Skills Questions (Professionalism, Research, Policy & Procedure, etc.)

- 11 Respiratory Therapy Fundamentals Questions (Airways, O2 therapy, etc.)

FORWARD

The practice of respiratory therapy entails pulling from diverse sets of knowledge from Mechanical Ventilation, Pathophysiology, and Cardiopulmonary Resuscitation etc. Understanding core concepts is not enough. To truly be proficient you must understand where sets of knowledge come together to influence the outcome. This is where you move from student to professional.

These questions have been identified as stumbling blocks, sometimes because of obscurity and sometimes because of the difficulty of the subject matter. In either case they still offer insight into the profession of respiratory therapy and this document offers you a chance to enhance your ability to become that professional.

As you review these problematic questions that have been identified by our database, study them with not only a view towards your exam but keeping in mind implications for your practice. Your career will and your patients will benefit greatly from paying attention to the little things.

Graham Werstiuk, RRT

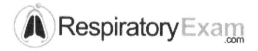

INTRODUCTION

I want to thank you for downloading *"The 66 Test Questions Respiratory Therapy Students Get Wrong Every Time…Volume 1 of 2"*

Volume 1 of 2 contains the 66 EXACT questions Respiratory Therapy Students keep getting wrong the most. They come from a large database comprising thousands of questions. Since you're reading this now, there is no reason that you will ever have to again.

To give you a little more background, our team built RespiratoryExam. com specifically for Student Respiratory Therapists, and its been running for a number of years now. The site has had excellent feedback from users, and during that time, we've had the chance to organize some VERY useful data.

The questions themselves are not very exciting, (unless you're a bunch of GEEKS like us) but when they do come up again, you can be certain you will get them correct, whether it is in class or quite possibly on your licensing exam.

NONE of the questions are sugarcoated. They're printed exactly as they are tested on students on RespiratoryExam.com, with a brief & short explanation at the end.

We really hope you find value in us publishing these questions, and we'll keep revising them periodically as change takes place. Stay tuned for a FREE BONUS at the end.

Thanks again for downloading this book, I hope you enjoy it!

Brady Nelson RRT

Patient Assessment

QUESTION 1:

Which of the following choices is most likely not associated with unilateral, decreased/absent, tactile fremitus?

a. Pneumothorax

b. Pleural Effusion

c. Atelectasis

d. Pneumonia

Correct Answer: d = Pneumonia

Explanation:

Tactile Fremitus is the transmission of vibration through the thoracic tissues. Transmission and the ability to feel this vibration will be increased in the setting of consolidation as seen with pneumonia. By comparison fluid and airspaces outside the lung will be comparatively poor conductors of vibration leading to reduced tactile fremitus. Atelectasis may also be a candidate but is less likely to be unilateral and is not the best answer in this question.

QUESTION 2:

Which of the following choices will affect the accuracy of pulse oximetry readings? 1) Motion artifact, 2) Intravascular dyes, 3) Fingernail polish, 4) Elevated serum bilirubin level, 5) Dark skin pigmentation.

    a.   1 and 5 only

    b.   1, 2 and 4

    c.   1, 2, 3 and 5

    d.   All of the above

Correct Answer: c = 1, 2, 3 and 5

Explanation:

Elevated serum bilirubin levels do not appear to affect pulse oximeter readings. Elevated levels in the blood result in a jaundiced appearance in the patient where the skin turns yellow in color but should not affect pulse oximetry especially when metabolically produced carbon monoxide is corrected for. The answer here is 1, 2, 3 and 5

QUESTION 3:

Carbon monoxide will have the following effects, except for..?

    a.   An oxygen dissociation curve left shift

    b.   A decrease in oxygen saturation measured by pulse oximetry

    c. SaO_2 measurement when calculated from ABG measurements

    d.   Decrease in PaO_2

    Correct Answer: d = Decrease in PaO_2

Explanation:

Recall that PaO_2 as measured is a reflection of the partial pressure of oxygen in the plasma. Even as carbon monoxide binds strongly to hemoglobin (explaining the effect on the other three options) there should be little change in PaO_2 unless oxygen is almost entirely depleted from the body.

QUESTION 4:

You have a female patient who has a history of liver failure and requires blood transfusions periodically. Her hemoglobin at the time of assessment is 125 g/dL.

You realize that her number is?

    a.   Erroneous

    b.   High

    c.   Low

    d.   Normal

Correct Answer: a = Erroneous

Explanation:

Your patient's hemoglobin at the time of assessment is 125 g/dL. You realize that her number is "Erroneous" due to the units. It should be in g/L, and with units as high as in the question, they are definitely in error. Normal range for hemoglobin in a female is 120 - 150 g/L. Therefore; the answer is "Erroneous"

QUESTION 5:

Methemoglobinemia is defined usually as a metHb concentration exceeding ____%?

a. 1-2

b. 3-5

c. 5-10

d. 15-20

Correct Answer: a = 1-2

Explanation:

At least some Methemoglobinemia is normal as a by product of metabolic and oxidative processes in the body. However this normal limit is typically below 1%. Therefore based on this conservative threshold any value above that would be considered pathological.

QUESTION 6:

The physician caring for your patient reports that the patient's cardiac output is 3.5 L/sec. You realize that this is _____?

a. Normal

b. High

c. Low

d. Erroneous

Correct Answer: d = Erroneous

Explanation:

Cardiac output should be reported in L/min. L/sec gives a value far too high. Note: if this was in L/min, 3.5 would be considered low as the normal is 4-8 L/min. Therefore, the answer here is "Erroneous"

QUESTION 7:

While performing chest percussion on your patient, you notice that your patient has a dull percussion note on the right lung only approximately 1cm above the right hemi-diaphragm. With resonance throughout the rest of the lung fields, and no increased work of breathing what do you most likely conclude?

a. A right sided pneumonia

b. A left sided pneumonia

c. A right sided effusion

d. Presence of the liver pushing up on the right hemi-diaphragm

Correct Answer: d = Presence of the liver pushing up on the right hemi-diaphragm

Explanation: The dull percussion note on the right lung palpated is due to the presence of the liver pushing up on the right hemi-diaphragm, and is normal.

QUESTION 8:

Unilateral pulmonary fibrosis will cause tracheal deviation..?

    a.   Toward the affected side

    b.   Away from the affected side

    c.   To shift posteriorly

    d.   To shift anteriorly

Correct Answer: a = Toward the affected side

Explanation: Unilateral pulmonary fibrosis would be exceedingly rare however this question tests your intuition around understanding the mechanisms. As the tissue tightens and shrinks on the affected side it will pull the mediastinum and related tissues towards the affected side. This assumes the pleura and pleural fluid are intact and functioning.

QUESTION 9:

Mixing of the arterial sample is most important for __ & __?

a. PaO2 & PaCO2

b. pH & Hb

c. pH & Hct

d. Hb & Hct

Correct Answer: d = Hb & Hct

Explanation: Mixing the sample won't have a huge effect on pH, PaCO2 or PaO2, but will effect hemoglobin and hematocrit measurement on the Co-oximeter. Therefore, the answer is "Hb & Hct"

QUESTION 10:

Which of the following conditions is most consistent with unilateral elevation of the left hemi-diaphragm? As pictured below.

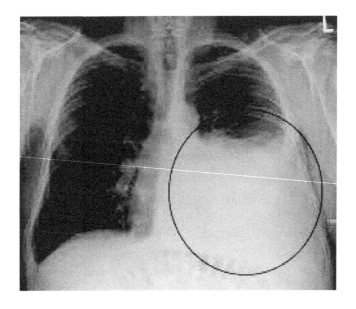

By James Heilman, MD (Own work) [CC BY-SA 3.0 (http://creativecommons.org/licenses/by-sa/3.0) or GFDL (http://www.gnu.org/copyleft/fdl.html)], via Wikimedia Commons

    a. COPD

    b. Asthma

    c. Pleural Effusion

    d. Pneumothorax

Correct Answer: c = Pleural Effusion

Explanation: COPD & Asthmatics would more often present with a bilateral process, which would be characterized by increased air space. Look to the right side of this xray. Typically with a pneumothorax, the x-ray would present with increased airspace (hyper-lucency). Although a pleural effusion can be bilateral, in this case it is unilateral and the fluid will always appear as increased density or "white" on an x-ray.

QUESTION 11:

Your patient has a CVP of 20 mmHg, there are many possible reasons for this.

Which of the following would not be one of them?

    a.   Right sided heart failure

    b.   Fluid Overload

    c.   Arterial thrombus

    d.   Positive airway pressure

Correct Answer: c = Arterial Thrombus

Explanation: Your patient has a CVP of 20 mmHg. First recognition should be made this is an abnormally high result. Arterial thrombus would not be a reason for this since central venous pressure is mostly affected in venous circulation if even due to a thrombus at all. Therefore, the answer here is "Arterial Thrombus". Normal CVP is from 3-8mmHg (5-10 cmH2O)

PULMONARY
FUNCTION

QUESTION 1:

1) Exhaled nitric oxide is experimentally used to titrate _____ in asthma?

    a.   Exercise

    b.   Beta Adrenergic medications

    c.   Corticosteroids

    d.   Anti-leukotrienes

    Correct Answer: c = Corticosteroids

Explanation:

Exhaled nitric oxide (eNO) is measured in a test for Asthma since NO is produced by specific cell types in the inflammatory response. Such small quantities are measured that parts per billion is used to quantify the eNO. In more recent years this has allowed us to titrate corticosteroids aimed at the inflammatory cascade in asthma.

QUESTION 2:

2) An increased occlusion pressure at 100 ms or 0.1 sec indicates
_____ drive to breathe?

    a.   an increased

    b.   reduced

    c.   an unchanged

    d.   None of the above

Correct Answer: a = an increased

Explanation:

An increased P100 or P 0.1 is thought to occur during an involuntary part of the breathing cycle. That is when there is an increase drive to breath the diaphragm will contract more forcefully regardless of voluntary effort during the first portion of the breath. This is reflected when a breathing circuit is briefly occluded during the first portion of the breath and this measurement is thought to positively correlate with drive to breath.

QUESTION 3:

3) What does a decrease in FEV1 indicate without change in FVC is an indication of?

 a. Obstructive changes

 b. Restrictive changes

 c. Mixed process

 d. Normal finding

Correct Answer: d = Obstructive changes

Explanation:

A change in FEV1 without concurrent decrease in FVC is characteristic of obstructive process. This decrease reflects impaired flow. This typically occurs due to airway narrowing and/or collapse. This finding can help aid in diagnosing asthmatic or COPD patients.

QUESTION 4:

4) The P100 is the most negative pressure a patient can generate against a closed circuit during the first one hundred milliseconds of a spontaneous effort. A normal P100 is _____?

    a.   15-20 cmH2O

    b.   10-15 cmH2O

    c.   6-10 cmH2O

    d.   2-4 cmH2O

Correct Answer: d = 2-4 cmH2O

Explanation:

A normal P100 is "2-4 cmH2O", which is therefore the answer. The P100 is the most negative pressure a patient can generate against a closed circuit during the first one hundred milliseconds of a spontaneous effort. The P100 value is indicative of the amount of neural activity that is causing diaphragm movement. The normal range is 2-4 cmH2O and a P100 < 6 cmH2O may be an indicator of readiness for weaning.

QUESTION 5:

5) A normal healthy patient of either gender should be able to generate a NIF (Negative inspiratory force) of at least?

    a. (-)20cmH2O

    b. (-)40cmH20

    c. (-)60cmH2O

    d. (-)100cmH2O

Correct Answer: c = (-)60cmH2O

Explanation:

In extubation guidelines often we only require patients to generate a NIF of – 20 or -25 cmH2O however this is a low threshold made for critically ill patients. A normal healthy patient of either gender should be able to generate a NIF of at least (-)60cmH2O and more likely can greatly exceed that threshold.

QUESTION 6:

6) Which phase of the single breath nitrogen washout test shows a sharp increase in the nitrogen and continues to the residual volume?

    a.   Phase 1

    b.   Phase 2

    c.   Phase 3

    d.   Phase 4

Correct Answer: d = Phase 4

Explanation:

The phase of the single breath nitrogen washout test shows a sharp increase in the nitrogen and continues to the residual volume is "Phase 4", which is therefore the answer. The start of phase 4 is called the closing volume (CV), marking the lung volume when small airway closure begins and also can be a marker of small airway disease.

QUESTION 7:

7) Which of the following is a lung volume or capacity is measured directly by spirometry, without use of specialized maneuvers or gases?

   a. VC

   b. FRC

   c. TLC

   d. RV

Correct Answer: a = VC

Explanation: The lung capacity that is not measured indirectly (it is measured directly) is vital capacity, or "VC", which is therefore the answer. VC can be obtained through direct spirometry. Other volumes and capacities require the use of measuring gases (helium and nitrogen) and specialized maneuvers.

QUESTION 8:

8) Closing Volume (CV) is expressed as a percentage of the Vital capacity (VC). In a young healthy adult the CV is equal to __% of the VC.

    a. 10

    b. 20

    c. 30

    d. 40

Correct Answer: a = 10

Explanation: Closing Volume (CV) is expressed as a percentage of the VC. In a young healthy adult the CV is equal to 10% of the VC. This is usually measured through a single nitrogen breath washout test, which can obtain both the closing capacity (CC) and closing volume (CV) in the lungs.

QUESTION 9:

9) The abbreviation for the amount of negative pressure generated at the mouth in the first 100 msec of inspiration against an occluded airway is?

    a. F0.01

    b. P0.01

    c. P100

    d. F100

Correct Answer: c = P100

Explanation: The abbreviation for the amount of negative pressure generated at the mouth in the first 100 msec of inspiration against an occluded airway is "P100", which is therefore the answer. The P100, also may be written as P0.1, measures of the neural output from the medullary centers that drive respiratory rate and volume. Normally, these pressures will increase with hypercapnia and hypoxemia.

QUESTION 10:

10) FEV1% is _____ with restrictive disease?

    a.   Decreased or normal

    b.   Increased or normal

    c.   Normal

    d.   Decreased

Correct Answer: b = Increased or normal

Explanation: Please note the % sign. This indicates the percentage of volume breathed out at 1 sec vs a volume or flow measurement. Due to the nature of most restrictive process compliance is severely decreased and the lungs want to return to resting state faster after inhalation. It would be expected then that the flow of gas relative to the total volume would be increased.

QUESTION 11:

11) Why is histamine sometimes used in place of methacholine?

    a.   It produces airway reactivity at a faster rate

    b.   Recovery of baseline function is faster

    c.   Histamine causes less damage to the airway

    d.   Methacholine action lasts for days

Correct Answer: b = Recovery of baseline function is faster

Explanation: Histamine is sometimes used in place of methacholine because the recovery of baseline function is faster. The nature of the receptor sites activated generally means that histamine will dissociate and be cleared sooner than methacholine. Although, histamine can cause nasal, bronchial mucus secretion and bronchoconstriction via the H1 receptor, while methacholine utilizes the M3 receptor for just for bronchoconstriction.

BASIC SCIENCE
FOR RESPIRATORY
THERAPISTS

QUESTION 1:

1) Which of the following is a characteristic of particles in a colloid?

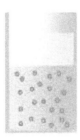

SunKart at en.wikipedia [CC BY 3.0 (http://creativecommons.org/licenses/by/3.0)], via Wikimedia Commons

a. Can not pass through filters or membranes

b. The solid settles out over time

c. Do not possess electrical charge

d. Are between 1-1000 nanometers in size

Correct Answer: d = Are between 1-1000 nanometers in size

Explanation:

A colloid refers to a liquid in which particles of another substance are indefinitely suspended within the liquid and do not dissolve. By convention when particles in a liquid mixture are less than 1000 nanometers but still greater than 1µm, they considered are colloids.

QUESTION 2:

2) End-tidal carbon dioxide monitoring (EtCO2), measures exhaled carbon dioxide using which technology?

    a. Spectrophotometry

    b. Mass spectrometer

    c. Polarographic analyzer

    d. Paramagnetic analyzer

Correct Answer: b = Mass spectrometer

Explanation:

End-tidal carbon dioxide monitoring is a technique by which exhaled carbon dioxide is measured by the use of a "Mass Spectrometer." Mass spectrometry is an analytical technique that produces spectra of the masses of the atoms or molecules comprising a sample of material.

QUESTION 3:

3) Which of the following is correct regarding atmospheric gases?

1. Carbon dioxide = 0.03%

2. Nitrogen = 70.01%

3. Nitrogen dioxide = 78.08%

4. Argon = 0.93%

5. Oxygen = 19.98%

a. 1 & 4

b. 2 & 5

c. 3 & 4

d. 1 & 2

Correct Answer: a = 1 & 4

Explanation:

Carbon dioxide = 0.03% & Argon = 0.93% are both correct.

QUESTION 4:

4) The type of compound formed when one atom gains an electron and one loses an electron is known as?

    a.   Covalent Compound

    b.   Molecular Compound

    c.   Positron Compound

    d.   Ionic Compound

Correct Answer: d = Ionic Compound

Explanation:

An "Ionic Compound" is formed when atoms transfer electrons, where one atom gives up an electron and another gains an electron. An example of this is NaCl.

QUESTION 5:

5) Which of the following reactions is a hydrocarbon + oxygen -->
carbon dioxide + water?

    a.   Decomposition

    b.   Combustion

    c.   Neutralization

    d. Nuclear

Correct Answer: b = Combustion

Explanation:

The breakdown of a hydrocarbon + oxygen, to carbon dioxide & water
is known as a "Combustion" reaction.

QUESTION 6:

6) Which law states the rate of diffusion of a gas is proportional to its concentration?

    a.   Boyle's Law

    b.   Fick's Law

    c.   Graham's Law

    d.   Henry's Law

Correct Answer: b = Fick's Law

Explanation:

"Fick's Law" states the rate of diffusion of a gas is proportional to its concentration. This law provides rationale for supplementing oxygen. We hope to influence diffusion by altering concentrations.

QUESTION 7:

7) Force per unit area is also known as?

    a.   Work

    b.   Pressure

    c.   Mass

    d.   Gravity

Correct Answer: b = Pressure

Explanation: Force / Area = "Pressure", which is therefore the answer.

QUESTION 8:

8) Which gas law states that the pressure of a gas of fixed volume is directly proportional to the gas' absolute temperature?

    a.   Gay Lussac's law

    b.   Henry's law

    c.   Daltons law

    d.   Charle's law

Correct Answer: a = Gay Lussac's law

Explanation: Gay Lussac's law states that the pressure of a gas of fixed volume is directly proportional to the gas' absolute temperature. The more practically a warmer gas will expand and a colder gas will contract. This provides the intuition behind a can of compressed contents exploding in a fire.

QUESTION 9:

9) This principle states that pressure drop across an obstruction can be restored if the angle of divergence is less than 15 degrees?

    a.   Bernoulli Principle

    b.   Venturi Principle

    c.   Archimedes' Principle

    d.   Constancy Principle

Correct Answer: b = Venturi Principle

Explanation: The "Venturi" principle states that pressure drop across an obstruction can be restored if the angle of divergence is less than 15 degrees. This applies when entraining room air through multiple devices in respiratory therapy.

QUESTION 10:

10) Which of the following are absolute zero scales?

1. Rankine

2. Celcius

3. Fahrenheit

4. Kelvin

    a. 1 & 2

    b. 2 & 4

    c. 1 & 4

    d. 3 & 4

Correct Answer: c = 1 & 4

Explanation: Of the given choices, the only two that are absolute zero scales are Rankine and Kelvin. Therefore, the answer here is "1 & 4". Absolute zero is considered the lowest temperature possible. -273.15 degrees Celsius and -459.67 degrees Fahrenheit coincide with 0 degrees Kelvin and 0 degrees Rankine.

QUESTION 11:

11) The capability of a system to maintain flow is known as?

    a. Conductance

    b. Resistance

    c. Velocity

    d. Gradient

Correct Answer: a = Conductance

Explanation: The capability of a system to maintain flow is known as "Conductance", which is therefore the answer. Conductance has an inverse relationship with resistance.

CARDIOPULMONARY ANATOMY & PHYSIOLOGY

QUESTION 1:

1) In a healthy patient's lungs, gas exchange is for the most part?

    a.   Greater in the bases

    b.   Greater in the apices

    c.   Greater in the mid-lung region

    d.   Unaffected by position

Correct Answer: a = Greater in the bases

Explanation:

Referring the principles of Ventilation and Perfusion matching. Blood flow and ventilation are most closely matched in the bases.

QUESTION 2:

2) The pressure measured as the difference between Pab - Ppl is _____?

    a.   Transabdominal Pressure (Pta)

    b.   Transesophageal Pressure (Ptes)

    c.   Transdiaphragmatic Pressure (Pdi)

    d.   Transpulmonary Pressure (Pl)

Correct Answer: c = Transdiaphragmatic Pressure (Pdi)

Explanation:

The pressure measured as the difference between Pab - Ppl is "Transdiaphragmatic Pressure (Pdi)", which is therefore the answer

QUESTION 3:

3) An alveolus that is ventilated but not perfused is referred to as _____ deadspace.

    a.   Physiologic

    b.   Alveolar

    c.   Anatomic

    d.   Mechanical

Correct Answer: b = Alveolar

Explanation:

An alveolus that is ventilated but not perfused is referred to as true alveolar deadspace. Therefore, the answer is "True alveolar" Alveolar deadspace may not even exist in normal persons, but due to V/Q mismatching can increase greatly in pulmonary diseases.

QUESTION 4:

4) The trachea begins at the ___ cervical vertebrate, to where it bifurcates at the carina at the ___ thoracic vertebrate.

    a. 4th, 5th

    b. 4th, 6th

    c. 5th, 7th

    d. 6th, 5th

Correct Answer: d = 6th, 5th

Explanation:

The trachea begins at the 6th cervical vertebrate, to where it bifurcates at the carina at the 5th thoracic vertebrate. Therefore, the answer here is "6th, 5th"

QUESTION 5:

5) A mountain climber ascends to 13,000ft.

During ascent which of the following factors does not decrease?

    a. $PaCO_2$

    b. PaO_2

    c. FiO_2

    d. Barometric Pressure

    Correct Answer: c = FiO_2

Explanation:

$PaCO_2$ will generally decrease due to hyperventilation secondary to a decrease in PaO_2 during ascent. As well Barometric pressure decreases during ascent, therefore the correct answer is "FiO_2", as FiO_2 stays constant near 21%.

QUESTION 6:

6) Which structures are the upper most and lower most points of the upper airway?

1. False Vocal Cords

2. True Vocal Cord

3. Posterior Nares

4. Anterior Nares

a. 1 & 2

b. 3 & 4

c. 1 & 3

d. 2 & 4

Correct Answer: d = 2 & 4

Explanation:

Simply by convention the highest point of the upper airway may be considered the anterior nares and the lower most point the true vocal chords.

QUESTION 7:

7) Total compliance of the respiratory system reflects total elastic resistance and _____?

    a.   Surface tension

    b.   Thoracic or Chest Wall (Cth)

    c.   Transdiaphragmatic Pressure (Pdi)

    d.   Transpulmonary Pressure (Pl)

Correct Answer: a = Surface tension

Explanation: Total compliance of the respiratory system reflects total elastic resistance and "Surface Tension." These are the forces that need to be overcome to provide ventilation.

QUESTION 8:

8) Which pressure is also known as intrathoracic pressure?

   a. Alveolar Pressure

   b. Intrapleural Pressure

   c. Esophageal Pressure

   d. Transpulmonary Pressure

Correct Answer: b = Intrapleural Pressure

Explanation: The pressure that is also known as intrathoracic pressure is intrapleural Pressure. By convention these both refer to the pressure within the pleural space.

QUESTION 9:

9) Where should the tip of a MacIntosh blade rest during when place fully into the airway?

    a.   Cricoid Cartilage

    b.   True Vocal Cords

    c.   Vallecula

    d.   Thyroid Cartilage

Correct Answer: c = Vallecula

Explanation: The tip of the Mac laryngoscope is placed into the "Vallecula" for the most optimal view, and is therefore the answer

QUESTION 10:

10) The trachea and large bronchi contain 3 distinct layers. Which is not one of those layers?

    a.   Cartilaginous layer

    b.   Mucoid Layer

    c.   Lamina propria

    d.   Epithelium

Correct Answer: b = Mucoid Layer

Explanation: The trachea and large bronchi contain 3 distinct layers. Those layers are the cartilaginous layer, the lamina propria, and the epithelium. The "Mucoid Layer" is not an actual tissue layer but refers only to the functional layer that forms when mucus and goblet cells are functioning.

QUESTION 11:

11) What are the names of the lateral borders of the nose?

    a.   Septum

    b.   Alae

    c.   Vestibule

    d.   Nasopharyx

Correct Answer: a = Alae

Explanation: The lateral borders of the nose are also known as "Alae."

SOFT SKILLS

(PROFESSIONALISM, RESEARCH, POLICY & PROCEDURE, ETC.)

QUESTION 1:

1) _____ relates to the ability of the test to identify those without the condition of interest.

    a. Specificity

    b. Sensitivity

    c. P-Value

    d. Population

Correct Answer: a = Specificity

Explanation:

Specificity relates to the ability of the test to identify negative results. The specificity of a test is defined as the group of patients who do not have the disease and test negative for it. Therefore, the answer is "Specificity".

QUESTION 2:

2) When doffing personal protective equipment (Mask, Gloves, Gown, Eye protection), how many times minimum should hand hygiene occur?

    a.   1

    b.   2

    c.   3

    d.   4

Correct Answer: b = 2

Explanation:

Doffing personal protective equipment (Mask, Gloves, Gown, Eye protection) should occur a minimum 2 times, in the order of Gloves, Gown, Hand Hygiene, Eye Protection, Mask, Hand Hygiene. Therefore, the answer here is "2"

QUESTION 3:

3) An infection control agent that will inhibit the growth and development of microorganisms without necessarily destroying them has which property?

    a. Bacteriocidal

    b. Bacteriostatic

    c. Virucidal

    d. Germicide

Correct Answer: b = Bacteriostatic

Explanation:

An agent that is bacteriostatic will inhibit further growth and reproduction but may not have the ability to actually kill a pathogen.

QUESTION 4:

4) Which of the following P-values, has no presumption against the null hypothesis?

    a.   P value less than 0.01

    b. $0.01 < \text{P-value} < 0.05$

    c. $0.05 < \text{P-value} < 0.1$

    d.   P value greater than 0.1

Correct Answer: d = P value greater than 0.1

Explanation:

By convention a P value of less than 0.05 we can reject the null hypothesis. A P value of 0.1 shows there is a good probability that this relationship could have happened by chance if the null hypothesis were true. Where typically the null hypothesis states there is no relationship between two variables.

QUESTION 5:

5) The _____ of a measurement system, also called reproducibility or repeatability, is the degree to which repeated measurements under unchanged conditions show the same results.

   a. Accuracy

   b. Precision

   c. Probability

   d. Validity

Correct Answer: b = Precision

Explanation:

Precision of a measurement system, also called reproducibility or repeatability, is the degree to which repeated measurements under unchanged conditions show the same results. Therefore, the answer here is "Precision"

QUESTION 6:

6) Specificity relates to the ability of the test to identify _____ results, within a clinical trial.

    a. Specified

    b. Standard

    c. True Positive

    d. True Negative

Correct Answer: d = True Negative

Explanation:

Specificity relates to the ability of the test to identify True Negative results. The specificity of a test is defined as the group of patients who do not have the disease and who test negative for it over those who test negative + false positives. More intuitively the probability of a negative test given that the patient is well.

QUESTION 7:

7) A good chemical disinfectant for home respiratory equipment cleaning is?

    a.   Quaternary ammoniums

    b.   Alcohols

    c.   Lodophors

    d. Acetic Acid

Correct Answer: d = Acetic Acid

Explanation: "Acetic acid" (Vinegar) is a good chemical disinfectant for home respiratory equipment cleaning because it is generally effective and is well tolerated for both materials of the equipment and the patients.

QUESTION 8:

8) Which of the following cleaning techniques is most appropriate for killing Haemophilus influenzae?

    a. Virucidal agents

    b. Bacteriocidal agents

    c. Bacteriostatic agents

    d. Sporicidal agents

Correct Answer: b = Bacteriocidal agents

Explanation: "Bacteriocidal agents" is then answer and will be most appropriate in killing Haemophilus influenzae since it is a bacteria and bacteriocidal agents kill all bacteria. Bacteriostatic agents will only prevent new bacterial growth.

QUESTION 9:

9) You begin monitoring your patient, and describe to the physician that they appear short of breath. Which part of your charting would this fall under?

a. Subjective

b. Objective

c. Assessment

d. Plan

Correct Answer: a = Subjective

Explanation: Because you are describing what your patient's chief complaint or state, this would fall under the subjective component of your charting. Objective component would include numbers or data, usually quantifying the patient's state. Assessment would include the differential diagnosis based on the subjective and objective information obtained. The plan would be what you are going to do next to treat the patient based on your assessment. Therefore, the answer here is "Subjective"

QUESTION 10:

10) What is the correct term when the researcher does not know the research participant's identity?

   a. Confidentiality

   b. Anonymity

   c. Sensitivity

   d. Blind

Correct Answer: b = Anonymity

Explanation: The correct answer is "Anonymity". Anonymity typically refers to the state of an individual's personal identity, or personally identifiable information, being publicly unknown.

QUESTION 11:

11) Sensitivity relates to the test's ability to identify _____ results, within a clinical trial.

    a. Specified

    b. Standard

    c. True Positive

    d. True Negative

Correct Answer: c = True Positive

Explanation: Sensitivity relates to the test's ability to identify "Positive" results. For example, if a test has high sensitivity than it is more likely to catch all those who are sick within a population but at the expense of more false positives. Stated another way sensitivity refers to the probability of a positive test given the disease is present.

RESPIRATORY THERAPY FUNDAMENTALS (AIRWAYS, O2 THERAPY, ETC.)

QUESTION 1:

1) All of the following are important endotracheal tube placement indicators, except?

    a.   Chest x-ray shows 4cm above the carina

    b.   End tidal carbon dioxide is 5mmHg

    c.   Bilateral breath sounds noted on auscultation

    d.   Decreased presence of gastric sounds

Correct Answer: b = End tidal carbon dioxide is 5mmHg

Explanation:

All of the following are important endotracheal tube placement indicators, except "End tidal carbon dioxide is 5mmHg", which is therefore the answer. An end tidal reading should be higher than 10mmHg to confirm placement, in the presence of adequate cardiac output. A reading this low could still be from the esophagus.

QUESTION 2:

2) Immediate potential complications with percutaneous tracheostomy tube insertion include?

1. Bleeding

2. Pneumothorax

3. Decreased LOC

4. Subcutaneous emphysema

a. 1, 2, & 3

b. 2, 3, & 4

c. 1, 3 & 4

d. 1, 2 & 4

Correct Answer: d = 1, 2 & 4

Explanation:

Immediate complications with percutaneous tracheostomy tube insertion can include bleeding, pneumothorax & subcutaneous emphysema. Therefore, the answer is "1, 2 & 4". In most cases, your patient would be fully sedated; therefore, decreased LOC is not a potential immediate complication.

QUESTION 3:

3) Which of the following is correct concerning the normal values of a P(A-a)O2 Gradient?

a. The gradient decreases with age

b. On 100% O2, every 50 mmHg difference in P(A-a)O2 approximates 10% shunt

c. Normal shunt < 20%

d. Primary hypoventilation can occur with a normal P(A-a)O2

Correct Answer: d = Primary hypoventilation can occur with a normal P(A-a)O2

Explanation:

Primary Hypoventilation and high altitudes are situations where hypoxemia can occur with a normal P(A-a)O2. Therefore, the answer is "Primary hypoventilation can occur with a normal P(A-a)O2".

QUESTION 4:

4) The Bourdon gauge flowmeter is not pressure compensated. Backpressure generated into the gauge when the flow is set at 8 L/min will cause the gauge to read?

a. The next step higher (On most 10 L/min)

b. Lower

c. The same flow as set

d. The next step lower (On most 6 L/min)

Correct Answer: c = The same flow as set

Explanation:

The Bourdon gauge is not pressure compensated. Backpressure generated into the gauge will say the gauge is reading higher than what the patient is actually receiving. Therefore, the answer is "The same flow as set". If backpressure causes the flow to drop to 4 L/min, the gauge will still read 8 L/min.

QUESTION 5:

5) Which phase of the cough is in response to afferent impulses, then the cough center stimulates inspiratory muscles?

    a. Irritation

    b. Inspiration

    c. Compression

    d. Expulsion

Correct Answer: b = Inspiration

Explanation:

The "Inspiration" phase of the cough is in response to afferent impulses, and then the cough center stimulates inspiratory muscles. Therefore, the answer is "Inspiration". This is the second phase and is closely followed by the compression phase.

QUESTION 6:

6) With a surgical tracheostomy, when should the first tube change take place?

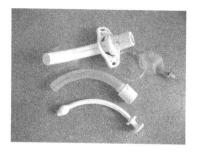

By Klaus D. Peter, Wiehl, Germany (Own work) [CC BY 2.0 de (http://creativecommons.org/licenses/by/2.0/de/deed.en)], via Wikimedia Commons

a. 1-3 days

b. 3-7 days

c. 7-10 days

d. 11-14 days

Correct Answer: c = 7-10 days

Explanation:

With a surgical tracheostomy, the first trach tube change should take place in "7-10 days", which is therefore the answer. This allows enough time for a stoma to develop and stabilize. The first trach tube change can take place 7 days post percutaneous tracheostomy, since the stoma site isn't as developed as a surgical trach.

QUESTION 7:

7) An LMA needs to have a cuff pressure of no more than ___ cmH2O.

    a. 30

    b. 45

    c. 60

    d. 75

Correct Answer: c = 60

Explanation: An LMA should have a cuff pressure of no more than "60" cmH2O, which is therefore the answer. Use of a manometer can decrease the prevalence of postoperative pharyngolaryngeal complications.

QUESTION 8:

8) In a Venturi mask, higher flow rates will cause?

    a.   Oxygen flow to drop to zero

    b.   FiO2 to decrease

    c.   FiO2 to increase

    d.   FiO2 to remain the same

Correct Answer: d = FiO2 to remain the same

Explanation: In the Venturi mask, a higher flow rate will cause the FiO2 to remain the same since proportional amounts of oxygen and air will always be entrained due to the venturi effect. Therefore, the answer is "FiO2 to remain the same".

QUESTION 9:

9) Of the following choices, humidity deficit is the difference between?

    a.   Room air and outdoors

    b.   Room air and 100% relative humidity

    c.   Room air and body humidity conditions

    d.   100% relative humidity and body humidity conditions

Correct Answer: c = Room air and body humidity conditions

Explanation: Humidity deficit is the difference between "Room air and body humidity conditions", which is therefore the answer. The humidity deficit is defined as the amount of water vapor that must be added to a gas in order to achieve 100% humidity at a specific temperature. The body must humidify all air entering the airways. If air enters the body and is 23C of 73F, even it is 100% relative humidity, it must be heated to 37C or 98F, then humidified to 100% relative humidity once again before entering the lower airways.

QUESTION 10:

10) To minimize complications from an NPA, it should be alternated between the left and right nares every _____.

    a.   4 hours

    b.   6 hours

    c.   12 hours

    d.   24 hours

Correct Answer: d = 24 hours

Explanation: To minimize complications from an NPA, it should be alternated between the left and right nares at least every "24 hours", which is a standard used in many hospitals. This can help prevent sinusitis and other nasal injury.

QUESTION 11:

11) Certain characteristics of hypertonic saline that the therapist should be aware of are?

1. It is a saline solution greater than 0.09%.

2. It is commonly used for sputum inductions.

3. Particles tend to shrink in size when nebulized.

4. A bronchodilator should be on hand when aerosolized hypertonic saline is used.

5. Samples for bacterial analysis should not be stored in hypertonic saline.

    a. I, II and IV

    b. I, II, and III

    c. II, IV, and V

    d. All of these are correct

Correct Answer: c = II, IV, and V

Explanation: Hypertonic saline is a solution greater than 0.9% and is commonly used for sputum inductions. Also, hypertonic saline particles tend to enlarge in size when nebulized, often require a bronchodilator be on hand when aerosolized, and should not be used to store samples for bacterial analysis. Therefore, the answer here is "II, IV, and V".

CONCLUSION

Thank you again for downloading this book!

I hope this book was able to help you to never get these specific questions wrong on any upcoming exams. Take these questions with a grain of salt. There was no bias in picking them, they are just the questions most continually answered incorrectly. Be sure that you will understand the concepts behind them to make sure you don't!

The next step is really just practice taking exams especially before your licensing exam, whether it's 1 or even 4 years down the road.

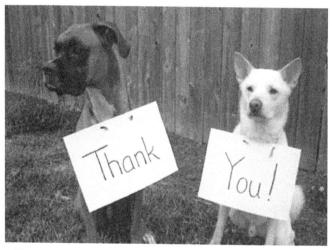

Finally, if you any feedback about the questions, please email us at info@respiratoryexam.com

Otherwise, I'd like to ask you for a favor, would you be kind enough to leave a review for this book? It'd be greatly appreciated!

Thank you and good luck!

Brady Nelson RRT

Made in United States
Orlando, FL
27 February 2022

15196307R00049